Title: 30 Days in James

A Devotional for Overcoming Addiction and Other Life-Altering Sins

By Dr. Brandon Bower, ThD, LCAC, CBAC

Published by Life Restoration Services

Categories: addiction, recovery, codependency, enabling, boundaries, restoration, faith, relationships

Paperback: 979-8-9908118-2-9

Ebook: 979-8-9908118-3-6

Contents

Introduction

In searching for a devotional for a friend who was caught in the throes of addiction, I realized that there were no great options.

I couldn't imagine that a devotional for addicts wasn't readily available. Having walked that journey over twenty-four years ago and having worked in the field of addiction for about that long, I realized that a devotional needed written and that I needed to write it. *30 Days in James* is the result.

It has been a great journey, and my prayer is that *30 Days in James* blesses you as you work through your addiction. May the following pages point you to the heavenly Father Who has the power to break the chains of addiction.

Day 1: A Servant of God

James 1:1 "James, a bondservant of God and of the Lord Jesus Christ, to the twelve tribes which are scattered abroad: greetings."

This is day one of your journey through the book of James. It starts with a big thought—the thought of being a servant of God.

When you think of the word *servant*, what comes to mind? I have never had or been a servant, at least in the traditional sense, so my mind goes to movies and TV series in which I have seen servants. *Batman*, *Downton Abby*, *The Brady Bunch* —these all had characters who served. But is this what James is talking about?

In this sense, James isn't calling himself a servant. He is literally calling himself God's slave. Well-known author and pastor John MacArthur put it this way: "The term servant as used in James refers to 'a person who is deprived of all personal freedom and totally under the control of his master.'"

Now, we understand what it means to be a slave. That's ultimately what addiction is, slavery to a substance. It may not start that way, but addiction always ends in slavery. Addiction is an awful experience. Based on our experiences with slavery to addiction, we don't ever want to experience that again!

It is a different type of scenario when James expresses that he is a slave to God than what we experienced with addiction. Being a bondservant of God starts with God. He is a loving Father Who has our best in mind. We are invited and welcomed to serve a God Who loves us abundantly, rescues us, and frees us unconditionally.

Daily Reflective Thoughts:

My Prayer: Lord, Heavenly Father,

Sincerely,

Day 2: Count It All Joy

James 1:2 "My brothers, count it all joy when you fall into various trials."

As addicts, there are many things that drive us, and the pursuit of happiness is often one of them.

Have you ever said, "I just want to be happy" either to someone or to yourself? The second verse of the book of James speaks into this pursuit. But instead of happiness, James tells us to be joyful. What's the difference?

Happiness is a pleasure, something to be felt, a reaction to something great. In Scripture, we are never called to pursue happiness. Joy, on the other hand, points us to Someone great. Why do we consider it joy when we face trials? Because while trials can steal your happiness, they can't steal your joy when your joy is found in Jesus. This may not make a lot of sense right away. This is probably because we, as Americans, are trained to seek happiness.

Let's look deeper into that. I often watch the lives of celebrities and famous people—those who seem to have it all. I watch their lives, actions, and struggles. They continue to pursue happiness even when it looks like they have everything anyone could ever want. But they are still empty. Joy, on the other hand, is a byproduct of a relationship.

If the Creator of the universe is my Master (see yesterday's lesson), then He knows my struggles, trials, urges, cravings, and hurts. He cares for me through them, guides me, directs me, and loves me unconditionally. This is why when we fall into various trials, we can be joyful. Try it, trust Him, and see how it changes you.

Daily Reflective Thoughts:

My Prayer: Dear Jesus,

Your child,

Day 3: When You Fall

James 1:2 "My brothers, count it all joy when you fall into various trials."

My dad is getting older.

Recently, he fell in the garage. He hit his shoulder pretty hard and suffered internal damage that hopefully time will heal. I called him shortly after and asked how he was doing.

"It hurts," was his reply. There is great truth in that little statement: falls hurt!

James knows this because he didn't say count it all joy if you *happen* to fall. He specifically said *when you fall.* Falls will happen. We will continue to sin, slip, and relapse. We live in a fallen world and, until Jesus returns, we will fall.

But there is hope! Because of Jesus's work on the cross, we don't have to stay down. That's where the joy part comes back in. Remember in yesterday's reading where we talked about how joy points us to Someone great? That is where our hope comes from—in the person and work of Jesus Christ.

Jesus didn't have to leave heaven and come to earth to **redeem** us. He didn't have to, but He wanted to!

Imagine: God's own Son stepped into the cosmos and came as a human baby. He lived among us, was tempted just as we are (see Hebrews 4:15) and remained sinless. He didn't fall! Even though He lived a perfect life, He chose to die as a perfect substitute for us (1 John 2:2) and pay the debt for all of our falls (sins). That's amazing news! That's where true joy comes from.

Definition of Redeem:

1. The action of saving or being saved from sin, error, or evil

2. The action of regaining possession of something in exchange for payment or clearing a debt

3. To buy back

The next time you fall, redirect your focus to the gift God has sent. Look up, get up, and keep going with joy!

Daily Reflective Thoughts:

My Prayer: Lord, thank you, Jesus,

Eternally grateful,

Day 4: Lack Wisdom – Ask God

James 1:5 "If any of you lacks wisdom, let him ask of God, Who gives to all liberally and without reproach, and it will be given to him."

The one thing I know about addiction is that abusing drugs/alcohol is poor judgment and shows a lack of wisdom.

Recovery is hard, very hard. Our bodies are used to the chemicals we were using, and withdrawal is painful, and sometimes almost impossible, to go through.

But another thing I know is that "if anyone lacks wisdom, let him/her ask of God" (James 1:5). God gives us wisdom wrapped in His unending grace! When we seek wisdom from God, He promises to provide it. He doesn't look at our mistakes, how many relapses we've had, or if we are worthy of His wisdom. He gives willingly to those who ask.

I think it's amazing that God doesn't look at our track record and judge whether or not we are worthy. Honestly, none of us is worthy, but He continues to give, and give, and give because He loves us. This is really good news! I personally am very grateful for His work in my life, saving me from myself, my struggles, my sins, and addictions. Thank God He didn't look at my track record!

So, when you are hurting, ask God. When you are struggling, ask God. When you have cravings, ask God. When you don't know what to do, ask God. When others are pushing you to do the wrong things, ask God for wisdom and help. He cares, and He always provides a way of escape (1 Corinthians 10:13), and wisdom to those who ask. So, ask!

Daily Reflective Thoughts:

My Prayer: Dear Lord,

Humbly asking,

Day 5: Nothing Wavering

James 1:6 "But let him ask in faith, with no doubting, for he who doubts is like a wave of the sea driven and tossed by the wind."

The King James Version of this verse says, "let him ask in faith, nothing wavering."

I like the way this version states it. What is **wavering?**

Definition of Wavering:

1. To sway to and fro; to flutter

2. To flicker or quiver

3. To shake and tremble; show doubt or indecision

In this verse, James is referring to asking for wisdom (see yesterday's devotional) while doubting that wisdom will actually be granted. Have you ever done this? I have. I remember a time when I asked God for help out of the mess I created and freedom from my sinful life. I needed help, but I didn't expect Him to answer. I thought I had to fix my own mess. I hadn't surrendered my life, and my heart was still focused on me.

We, as addicts, often waver, being driven to and fro by the storms in our lives. Several years ago, I went shark fishing with my brother and a few other family members. But I didn't anticipate being seasick. We were several miles out in the Atlantic Ocean, and our little fishing boat was wavering to and fro on the open sea. My body went berserk—I was dizzy, lightheaded, and puked several times.

When your life is out of control, body going berserk, and you're tossed to and fro, He is the anchor in your storm. Ask the God of the universe for wisdom in faith, not wavering, and He will help. It's His unbreakable promise to you. Turn to Him, turn your heart over to Him, and let Him have control. It's the best decision you will ever make.

Daily Reflective Thoughts:

My Prayer: Dear Savior,

Without wavering,

Day 6: A Doubleminded Man is Unstable

James 1:8 "he is a double-minded man, unstable in all his ways."

I was seriously unstable. I had been kicked out of college twice, arrested, and not trusted by those who loved me. Addiction tends to do that. Can you relate?

When James says a **double-minded** man is unstable in all his ways, he really means all of one's life—the whole of it. But look at the promise in Isaiah 26:3: "You will keep him in perfect peace whose mind is stayed on You."

Unstable versus perfect peace—it's not a hard choice, but hard to make happen. Why is it so hard to do what is right? Why is it so hard to keep our minds turned toward the Savior? The answer lies in where your heart is.

Definition of Double-Minded:

1. Wavering in mind; undecided

2. Marked by hypocrisy; insincere

Matthew 6:24 talks about how no one can serve two masters but will be loyal to one over the other. A double-minded man wants to love God and still have the pleasures of the world. For example, "I can use mind-altering substances and still love and worship God, right?" I have had these double-minded thoughts, too.

So, what steps help keep our mind focused on the Savior? First, you have to know Him. Not just know of Him, but truly know Him. That process starts with a willing heart.

The next step is to seek Him. The best place to start seeking the Savior is in His book, the Bible. Scripture tells us that if we seek Him, we will find Him.

Finally, turn your life over to His care. This is best done with a mentor; someone who can help you see your double-mindedness and keep pointing you toward the Savior. Do you have someone like this in your life? If not, ask God to send you one.

I found perfect peace through a personal relationship with Jesus. I challenge you to do the same.

Daily Reflective Thoughts:

My Prayer: Hey God,

Seeking You,

Day 7: Endure Temptation = Blessed

James 1:12
"Blessed is the man who endures temptation; for when he has been approved, he will receive the crown of life which the Lord has promised to those who love Him."

Blessed.

I wanted that, I sought that, but I never found it in my mess. My addiction took control, took the blessings from my life.

Now, today, I am blessed. Blessing comes through enduring temptation. The key here is having complete trust in the Savior, passing through the trials of temptation with your faith in Christ still solid. The man or woman who does this has God's approval and true salvation.

It's time to talk about true salvation. I was taught as a kid to say a prayer and that God would live in my heart and I would be free from the threat of Hell. A magic prayer—who wouldn't want that? That's false teaching, it is a devastating lie that is damning many to Hell. Salvation comes through placing our complete trust in our Savior. This may start as a prayer, but it doesn't end there! Please read the addendum at the back of this book titled *An Explanation of the Gospel.*

If you have never experienced true salvation, please contact us (see our contact information at the end of this book). We want you to experience the true and lasting peace that can only be found through a personal relationship with God. We want you to have a blessed life - a life controlled by the Savior, not your addiction.

Daily Reflective Thoughts:

My Prayer: Here in my life,

Humbly asking,

Day 8: Drawn Away

James 1:14 "But each one is tempted when he is drawn away by his own desires and enticed."

Yup, we understand this verse because it explains addiction perfectly!

Every human is tempted. We are not special because we use/used alcohol and drugs. Our inner desire to satisfy our heart's longings has dragged us into the trap of sin. It happened to me, and I was in deeper than I ever planned. Sadly, sometimes I am enticed to return to my dark desires. Our temptations are a symptom of a deeper heart problem.

Sin is attractive. That's the trap of addiction. If it wasn't pleasurable, our hearts wouldn't seek it. But like any well-planned trap, the pleasure only lasts until we are caught, stuck, or unable to escape. It is entirely our fault when we choose to return. We know better, but we let our hearts wander back into the mess. Can you relate?

This is why we are told in Scripture to guard our hearts (Proverbs 4:23). Protecting our hearts is a full-time job, and we need all the help we can get. That's why mentors are important. They can often see things we can't. The problem is we are too embarrassed to share our struggles. So, we keep them inside, protecting them from the world, and secretly visit them when no one is looking.

But God sees what's in our hearts. We can't hide our struggles and sin from Him. But we can ask for His help. He promises to help if we ask (Matthew 7:7). Have you sought help? Do you have support to help you guard your heart from temptation and your heart's sinful desires? Asking for help is healthy and a necessary step in our recovery if we want to truly change.

Daily Reflective Thoughts:

My Prayer: Lord, help me,

Needing You,

Day 9: Desire → Sin → Death

James 1:15
"Then, when desire
has conceived, it
gives birth to sin;
and sin, when it
is full-grown, brings
forth death."

Sin follows a simple process: the lusts (desires) in our hearts —> birth sin in our lives —> which leads to poor choices and bad decisions —> which leads to death.

The process is devastating and leads to eternal separation from God in a place called Hell (eternal death). But the sin process can be stopped! To do this, we have to start with the lust in our hearts.

That little pet sin—you know, the one you have been holding on to for years, the one you hide from everyone, the one you turn to when the pressures of life weigh down your soul—this is the sin that I want to talk about. It is born of a heart desire and if left unchecked, it will grow into a monster.

Maybe it already has. This pet sin is enough to separate you from God for all eternity. Think about that. Is it worth it?

The way out is another simple process: **Confess** —> Repent —> Turn! To confess means to admit or state that one has committed a crime or is at fault in some way. Scripture is clear that if we confess our sins, God is faithful and just to forgive us our sin and to cleanse us from *all* unrighteousness (I John 1:9).

I have a friend who loved his little pet sin. He turned to it often, and it was destroying his family. He would get caught and be quick to "confess," but there was no turning.

Confession without turning isn't true heart change.

Definition of Confess:

1. Admit or state that one has committed a crime or is at fault in some way

2. To declare

Here is where we stop to think about turning - turning from sin, turning toward our Savior, and not turning back. Ask for help with this process; then do it.

You won’t regret it!

Daily Reflective Thoughts:

My Prayer: Lord, I confess,

Turning it over,

Day 10: Good Gifts from the Father

James 1:17 "Every good gift and every perfect gift is from above, and comes down from the Father of lights, with whom there is no variation or shadow of turning."

I remember my 4th grade birthday party very well.

I invited Ben. I didn't like Ben much, but his mom always bought the best gifts. Not only were they super nice, they were wrapped well with colorful paper, perfectly curled ribbon, and balloons. There were always balloons. So, Ben was invited to my party.

The big day came, and all my friends showed up, except Ben. I waited and waited. Finally, he ran in late with a plastic Walmart bag. He threw it on the table and joined the others. I was devastated. No fancy wrapped gift. I felt unloved, unwanted, and I'm sure I cried.

Ben's mom, forgetting about the party and running late that day, stopped at Walmart and picked up something. It was a big letdown. I don't even remember anything I got for my 4th grade birthday party, but I remember feeling unloved because of that gift.

James tells us that every good gift is from God. My friend, if you have a good gift, make sure you thank God for it! Thank Him for family, sobriety, peace, sunshine, the water you drink, and the air you breathe. Thank Him for the gift of His one and only Son who came to Earth, lived a sinless life, died a sinless death, and took the penalty of your sin to set things right between you and God. That, my friend, is a perfect gift given to you by your Father in Heaven who deeply loves and cares for you.

Daily Reflective Thoughts:

My Prayer: Thank you for the gift of,

Eternally grateful,

Day 11: Swift to Hear

James 1:19 "So then,
my beloved brethren,
let every man be
swift to hear, slow to
speak, slow to wrath."

I noticed something when I turned forty—my hearing (as well as many other things) didn't work as well as it used to.

If there is any background noise at all, I have trouble hearing. My wife can attest to this, and she would probably tell you it happened many years earlier… but I noticed it at forty.

James is talking to the child of God in today's verse, one who claims to be a Christ follower and shows his/her faith through his/her actions. His first piece of advice is to be swift to hear. Swift to hear what? The Word of God!

You can't hear what God is saying if you don't read His book. Hebrews 4:12 tells us that God's Word is "living and powerful," helping guide us through this life. But are you listening? God wants to teach you though His Word. He wants to talk to you and be your friend.

So, listen. I recommend getting a study Bible, one with notes and commentary that can help you better understand what you are reading. It's amazing what we learn, how we grow, and how quickly we can change if we actually listen and understand what God is telling us.

Check out the *Resource Page* at the back of this book for recommendations on a study Bible and other materiel that can help you on your journey with Christ.

Daily Reflective Thoughts:

My Prayer: As I am listening,

Teach me,

Day 12: Slow to Speak

James 1:19 "So then,
my beloved brethren,
let every man be
swift to hear, slow to
speak, slow to wrath."

We all know that person who never stops talking—like, never. It's annoying, frustrating, and shows their ignorance.

It is told that a man came to Socrates to be an intern and learn from one of the wisest men around. The man talked for ten minutes about his status, the people he knew, how he was a great student, and how he would be a great learner. After the man was done, Socrates said he would take on the intern but would have to charge him double what the other interns paid. The man was perplexed and asked why.

Socrates answered, "I first have to teach you how to shut your mouth, then I have to teach you how to use it."

Scripture talks often about the value of being slow to speak. Proverbs 13:3 says, "Whoever guards his mouth preserves his life; he who opens wide his lips comes to ruin." How can you be swift to hear if you can't hear over the ramblings of your mouth?

There is a counseling tool I often use in my life. It helps with my decision making and allows me to be slow to speak. When someone asks me something that I am unsure about, I haven't thought about, or that I am uncomfortable with, I tell them that I need to take a moment to process their request, and I will get back to them later in the day. This allows me to not get trapped into doing something I don't want to do or from answering before I have thought through the matter.

I challenge you to take some time and reflect on the wisdom you see in James here.

Daily Reflective Thoughts:

My Prayer: As I ponder,

With thoughtful response,

Day 13: Slow to Anger

James 1:19 "So then,
my beloved brethren,
let every man be
swift to hear, slow to
speak, slow to wrath."

Years ago, I owned a blue Chevy S-10 pickup truck. It was a rocking truck, which I enjoyed more than any other vehicle I have owned.

One day, I went to the store for my wife to buy diapers and milk for our young son. After I was finished shopping, I returned to my truck to find that someone had smashed into it and dented the tailgate really bad. In my extreme anger (**wrath**), I reacted. I threw the milk on the ground and scanned the parking lot to see if I could find the evildoer who had destroyed my truck. I pulled out my keys and tried to get into the truck, but to no avail. The lock was jammed. My anger raged even more!

Define Wrath:

1. Extreme anger

2. Rage, fury, indignation

Then it happened. I saw a hula girl figurine dancing on my dashboard. I didn't have a hula girl on my dashboard. My heart sank in embarrassment. It wasn't my truck. My truck was three aisles over and as perfect as I had left it. I made a fool of myself that day. I'm sure it was a funny sight. And oh, how I dishonored by Savior in my anger. I think of that day often and what I learned.

James's third piece of advice to the Christ-follower is to be slow to wrath or anger. Check yourself, slow down, and evaluate the situation before you slam the milk jug onto the parking lot pavement. Don't let your anger destroy your testimony and reputation.

Daily Reflective Thoughts:

My Prayer: As I confess my anger,

With sorrow,

Day 14: Put Away All Filthiness

James 1:21 "Therefore lay aside all filthiness and overflow of wickedness, and receive with meekness the implanted Word, which is able to save your souls."

I remember the day my preteen boys returned from their first week of summer camp.

They were excited, had a wonderful time, and smelled horrendous. That night, my wife described the laundry. One half of their packed clothing had not been worn, and the other half needed to be taken out and burned. They wore what they wanted and didn't shower as much as they should have. They were filthy.

Just like the boys needed to change their filthy clothes and put on new clothes after a long shower, we are to put off our old filthy behavior and put on new actions. In today's verse, James is talking about **moral failure** and tells us to change. Moral failure is doing wrong, sinning, committing wickedness, and going against moral values.

In the last part of that verse, James says "receive with meekness the implanted Word, which is able to save your souls." He didn't say put off old behavior or do better. Scripture says we can't save our own souls by "works of righteousness" or good works.

Our souls are saved by the implanted Word of God, the Bible. Not just knowing what He says, but by it being planted deep in our being. There is a big difference.

Definition of Moral Failure:

1. Wrong behavior; going against moral values

2. Sin, wrongdoing, wickedness

Take some time to talk to God about having His Word planted deep in your heart. Ask Him to help with this. By His work in your life, and the gift He gave through sending His Son, you can find freedom for your soul.

Daily Reflective Thoughts:

My Prayer: I deeply need You, Lord,

Seeking help,

Day 15: Keep Yourself Unspotted

James 1:27 "Pure and undefiled religion before God and the Father is this: to visit orphans and widows in their trouble, and to keep oneself unspotted from the world."

When I first was exposed to recovery talk, I was told I needed to change my people, places, and things.

They said this would help me avoid temptation and the chance of relapse.

Then I was to do service work to keep myself busy.

This was great, but there was something missing—the part about changing my heart.

My actions were in the right place, but my heart wasn't. I would show up, do service work, and proudly announce to everyone what *I was doing*. I was keeping myself sober and clean. I missed the part of humility and of letting God change my heart, soul, and mind.

I didn't have pure motives or undefiled or unspotted actions. They were still one hundred percent selfish!

My heart didn't demonstrate a true sacrificial love for others or for God. It's all about the heart change because true change starts there!

As you ponder this passage in James, I wonder if you (as I did) are doing good things from selfish heart motives?

Take a look at Matthew 15:19 where we see the heart is the place where evil thoughts, murder, adultery, sexual immorality, theft, false witness, and **slander** originate. If you want to keep yourself clean, check in on your heart motives.

Definition of Slander:

1. **The action or crime of making false state-**

ments

2. Damaging a person's reputation with lies

Daily Reflective Thoughts:

My Prayer: Father, as I evaluate my heart,

Needing You,

Day 16: Guilty = Offend in Only One Point

James 2:10 "For whosoever shall keep the whole law, and yet offend in one point, he is guilty of all."

My son got a Rokr clock puzzle for Christmas, a clock that you build out of wood.

There are hundreds of wood gears, and it is a pretty precise piece of machinery. He did an amazing job putting all the gears in the correct spot and building an awesome looking clock. He was so proud of his work. The time came to turn it on and see it run.

But it didn't. He wasn't sure what was wrong. He had spent hours on it. He later realized one of the first pieces he installed, a small piece, was off by just a tiny amount. As a result, he had to tear the whole thing apart just to fix the one piece that was installed wrong.

James uses a similar illustration when he talks about keeping the whole law but slipping just once. He says that one thing out of place ruins the way it's supposed to work. Scripture tells us in Ecclesiastes 7:20 that "there is not a righteous man on earth who does good and never sins."

We all have sinned; we all have offended in at least one way. Thus, we are **guilty** of all.

Definition of Guilty:

1. Responsible for wrongdoing

2. A standing of guilt

The amazing part of this whole mess is that God is in the process of redeeming guilty people. We are all guilty, we all need saving, and we all have been given the chance to seek forgiveness from Him. Have you turned your will and your life over to the care of Jesus?

Because of His sinless life and what He did for us through His death and resurrection, He can forgive us our sins and cleanse us from all unrighteousness. He removes our guilty status and replaces it with the title Child of God. What an amazing change in status!

Daily Reflective Thoughts:

My Prayer: Rejoicing in Him,

Thank you, Jesus,

Day 17: Lusts That War Inside

James 4:1 "Where
do wars and
fights come from
among you?
Do they not come from
your desires
for pleasure that
war in your
members?"

In 1984, the hit movie *Terminator* starring Arnold Schwarzenegger came out.

The film was a fan favorite where good and evil battle. In the movie, one of the key characters says, "Listen and understand. That terminator is out there. It can't be bargained with, it can't be reasoned with, it doesn't feel pity or remorse or fear. And it absolutely will not stop, *ever*, until you are dead!"

Does it sound familiar? I think it describes addiction perfectly.

The fight of your life starts with the lust in your heart. This quietly grows, larger and larger, until it seems uncontrollable. Just like the Terminator, lust is out there. It can't be bargained with, it can't be reasoned with, and it doesn't feel pity or remorse or fear. And it absolutely will not stop until you are dead. But there is a Savior!

We are told in Scripture to put to death the lusts of the heart (Colossians 3:5-6). We do this purposefully with the help of the Savior. We can't do it alone; we need help.

Those who have claimed Christ as their Savior have a secret weapon in the fight against the lusts of the heart. It is the Holy Spirit, given to guide and help us, Who **intercedes** for us as we enter the fight of our life! He has been given to us to be our guide and helper. What an amazing gift!

Definition of Intercede:

1. To intervene on behalf of another

2. To pray for

Don't back down. It's a fight you have to win, and it starts by fighting against the lusts of your heart.

Daily Reflective Thoughts:

My Prayer: Lord, as I fight my lust,

Thank You for fighting for me,

Day 18: You Have Not Because You Ask Not

James 4:2 "You lust, and have not: you kill, and desire to have, and cannot obtain: you fight and war, yet you have not, because you ask not."

God wants you, even welcomes you, to ask Him for help fighting this war of addiction.

Check out what is said in John 16:24: "Until now you have asked for nothing in My name; ask and you will receive, so that your joy may be made full." Ask God for the good things, to help with the hard things, and most importantly to work in your heart to change you. Asking is a prescription for joy.

Paul E. Miller wrote in his book *A Praying Life*, "**Prayer** is asking God to get dirty in your life. Yes, the eternal God scrubs floors. For sure we know He washes feet. So, take Jesus at His word. Ask Him. Tell Him what you want. Get dirty.

Write out your prayer requests; don't mindlessly drift through life on the American narcotic of busyness. If you try to seize the day, the day will eventually break you. Seize the corner of His garment and don't let go until He blesses you. He will reshape the day."

Definition of Prayer:

1. A request for help

2. An act of asking God

Asking for help, especially help from the Creator of the universe, is often hard to do. It's hard for humans, hard for addicts, hard for sinners. Hard, but good! While we toil and struggle in our mess, sometimes the best thing that we can do is stop and ask, let it go, and trust the God Who made you and me. He's got this; now move on.

Take some time to stop today and talk to God. Let Him inside the ugliness, and He will begin the healing process.

Daily Reflective Thoughts:

My Prayer: As I struggle to ask,

Thanks for listening,

Day 19: Enemies of God

James 4:4 "You adulterous people! Do you not know that friendship with the world is enmity with God? Therefore, whoever wishes to be a friend of the world makes himself an enemy of God."

Beyond a shadow of doubt, I know there is one thing I do not want to be—and that's an enemy of God! God, the Creator of the universe, the world that we live in, will win in any war I raise against Him. There is no winning that fight.

I doubt that any of us really sees ourselves as the enemy of God. You may think that you and God are friends, or you acknowledge He exists, or you are pleasant toward Him, or you go to church on occasion. But for sure, you are not enemies. James sees it differently and asks an important question: "Are you friends with the world or with God?" You can't be both.

What does it mean to be friends with this world? It all goes back to heart issues. Do I have a longing to follow God and His direction, or is my heart pulled to the attractions of this world? Money, lust, cars, power, and the list goes on. Where do the affections of your heart rest?

We often skew this by creating a god of our own understanding. We can love a god we create. Take the good, add a little bit, allow things we want, and behold! You have created a god who fits your desires. This, my friends, is idol worship and makes you the enemy of the one true God.

Check out 1 John 2:15 as it also has a lot to say about this subject. What idols might you be holding on to?

Daily Reflective Thoughts:

My Prayer: As I look at my longings,

Seeking You,

Day 20: God Resists the Proud

James 4:6 "But He gives more grace. Therefore, He says: God resists the proud, but gives grace to the humble."

C. S. Lewis, in his book *Mere Christianity*, said this about pride: "A proud man is always looking down on things and people; and, of course, as long as you are looking down, you cannot see something that is above you."

Some say that pride was the first sin, the sin that is at the root of all other sin. I don't disagree. If pride has you looking down, you are first and foremost missing a relationship with God. A heart full of pride isn't focused on Christ. I would also contend that a prideful heart is missing out on relationships with others.

James addresses pride here in this passage and goes one step further than C. S. Lewis. James says that those who harbor pride in their hearts - the self-centered, the defiant - are in conflict with God. We talked before about not wanting to be God's enemy, and pride is another way we set our hearts against God. The proud have no part of God's grace and are of no use in God's kingdom.

However, God gives grace to the **humble**. Take a deeper look into Matthew 5 when it says, "Blessed are the poor in spirit (humble) for theirs is the kingdom of God." Compare that passage to Proverbs 6, where God talks about his hatred of the proud, defiant sinner's sinful heart. In doing this comparison, we see a glimpse of God's heart and care for us. He wants us to reject pride, live a humble life, and seek Him with all our heart.

Definition of Humble:

1. A modest view of one's importance

2. Freedom from pride; not arrogant

What would it look like for you to have a humble heart that follows after God?

Daily Reflective Thoughts:

My Prayer: Help me put aside,

Humbly,

Day 21: Submit, Draw Near, Resist the Devil

James 4:7-8 "Therefore submit to God. Resist the devil and he will flee from you. Draw near to God and He will draw near to you."

This passage may be easy to understand—the steps are simple. But it isn't easy to live out, especially consistently.

You cannot be saved without submitting yourself to God and purposefully coming under His sovereign authority as Lord. What sounds easy here requires heart surgery, cutting away pride and sin in our hearts and replacing it with a love for Christ.

James then goes on to say that not only do we need to submit to God, but we also need to resist the Devil. Resist means to stand against or to oppose. The Devil is the author of lies, the deceiver of souls, and the manipulator of truth. There is great freedom in resisting him!

Resisting is a personal task, but being a part of a team helps greatly. Who on your team can help you in the resisting process? A mentor, friend, pastor, spouse, or counselor? Rely on these people when you are struggling. Allow them into the depths of your heart and let them come alongside you in this fight.

Next, James gives us a clue on how to submit and resist, which is best done by applying the third command of this passage: draw near to God. This means coming into deep fellowship with the God Who loves you and wants the best for you.

Compare that to the works of the Devil, and it's an obvious choice. But a choice it is!

Which will you choose?

Daily Reflective Thoughts:

My Prayer: Help me draw near,

Following You,

Day 22: Cleanse Your Hands

James 4:8 "Draw near to God, and He will draw near to you. Cleanse your hands, you sinners, and purify your hearts, you double-minded."

When James talks about cleansing our hands, he is referring to coming under the guidance of and submitting to Jesus.

This instruction is specifically directed to those who do not have a personal relationship with Him.

First John 1:9 says, "If we confess our sins, He (Jesus) is faithful to forgive us our sins and to cleanse us from all unrighteousness." The word *cleanse* here in

1 John 1:9 has the same meaning as it does in James. The only way to cleanse your hands is though Jesus.

Think about it this way: have you ever tried washing dishes with a dirty, filthy rag? The dish may look somewhat better, but you wouldn't eat off of it. You need a clean rag, one that isn't dirty.

The same goes with cleansing your life. Sinners can't cleanse their own hearts. We need Someone Who has never sinned to do that for us. That is the simple truth of the gospel. Gospel means good news and the good news is that Jesus Christ has already done the work for us that cleanses our hearts.

Turn your will and your life over to Jesus's care and let Him cleanse you of your sins. Trust in His eternal plan and start living a changed life! It's only through Him that you can find freedom.

Daily Reflective Thoughts:

My Prayer: Lord, I surrender,

Desperate for You,

Day 23: Purify Your Hearts

James 4:8 "Draw near to God, and He will draw near to you. Cleanse your hands, you sinners, and purify your hearts, you double-minded."

Did you know that all sin starts in the heart?

In this passage, James is linking the sins of our hands with the sins of the heart. Matthew 15:19 states that out of the heart comes every evil thing. We live in a world that says to "follow your heart, trust your heart, rely on your heart." God's response to that is a firm no! Throughout Scripture, we are reminded to guard our heart, guide our heart, protect our heart, and never to trust our heart.

I have a farmer friend who raises pigs. She often gives those pigs baths, but guess what? They always return to the mud pit. How true of our hearts as well.

Part of purifying your heart is to not dirty it again by doing the same things you were doing before. Call it relapse, a slip, or returning to your sin, it's all the same thing. The sin that so easily traps us can have no place in our hearts or lives!

Repentance, the act of totally turning the opposite way of sin, is the tool God uses to purify our hearts. Repentance is what brings new intentions, habits, and desires. God and God alone knows your heart, what you think, and your plans and purposes. Even the hardest of hearts can be transformed by the Savior.

May you have the freedom of a purified heart and the strength through the power of Christ to keep it that way!

Daily Reflective Thoughts:

My Prayer: Keep my heart clean,

Trusting You,

Day 24: Humble Yourself

James 4:10 "Humble yourselves before the Lord, and He will exalt you."

Exalting ourselves is a huge problem in our culture today.

We think "I've got this," or "I'm smart enough to do this on my own." But what draws God to us is not our goodness (we don't have any); it's our desperate need for help.

God loves us so much that He stepped out of heaven to rescue us! Our response to this is one of humility—to be humble enough to realize that He alone can fix this mess and that He alone deserves the glory for it.

Take a look back at James 4:6: "God is opposed to the proud but gives grace to the humble." Our humility needs to be seen in that we are completely unworthy because of our sin. To think that we can save ourselves sets us in opposition to Christ.

When we seek to have a clean, pure heart, it starts with the acknowledgement of our sin, our unworthiness, and His worthiness and ability to do something about it. What a gift!

Daily Reflective Thoughts:

My Prayer: Lord, it's time to let You,

Letting You in,

Day 25: Life is a Vapor

James 4:14b "What is your life? For you are a vapor that appears for a little time and then vanishes."

I have lived in some amazing places—Chicago, West Virginia, Austria, and most recently Indiana. I enjoy traveling, driving, and seeing the world God has created.

But there is one thing that I hate, and that's fog (in Chicago it's called smog). Fog is dangerous, blocks the view, and is an overall nuisance. James is stating in today's verse that our life is like that foggy night—uncertain, obscure, and quick to end.

J. Vernon McGee once wrote, "Human life lived apart from and without God is the most colossal failure in God's universe. Everything else serves a long and useful purpose. Human life apart from God is out of joint, dislocated, a colossal failure."

We do not control our lives. Our lives are solely in the hands of God.

Because of the brevity of life, why do we spend our time in jealousy, anger, discontent? These things spoil life.

An abundant life happens when we come before Christ and surrender our will and our lives to Him and His purpose for us. This is when we really start living!

Are you living that kind of life?

Daily Reflective Thoughts:

My Prayer: Surrender is hard, Lord. Here is what I need to lay down,

Living transparently,

Day 26: Yes...Yes, No...No

James 5:12 "But above all, my brothers, do not swear by heaven or by earth or by any other oath, but let your 'yes' be yes and your 'no' be no, so that you may not fall under condemnation."

It's quite a shame that people lie. It causes hurt, distrust, and pain, and is not easily reconciled.

By nature, we are liars. This is no surprise as Satan is the father of lies (John 8:44). This dishonesty has led to disaster, so man tries to fix it with new laws, rules, and treaties. These are all a result of our lying nature.

As James starts concluding his letter, he tells us that when we say we will do something, to keep our promise. It also says that when you say no, or promise to not do something, don't waver. All words matter, all words have consequences, and all our words will someday be judged by God. When we lie, we trample on the greatness and dignity God placed in all humans.

Proverbs 18:21 warns us that life and death are in the power of the tongue. Let your yes be yes and your no be no is a simple thought to take seriously—as seriously as though you were standing in a courtroom testifying before the Judge of the universe, because you are! All of our conversations should be guided by this principle.

Remember, every word that proceeds out of your mouth starts in the heart! Guard your heart.

Daily Reflective Thoughts:

My Prayer: Jesus, I need help with my words, please,

Changing daily,

Day 27: Pray, Sing, Call

James 5:13-14 "Is anyone among you suffering? Let him pray. Is anyone cheerful? Let him sing praise. Is anyone among you sick? Let him call for the elders of the church, and let them pray over him, anointing him with oil in the name of the Lord."

Are you suffering? The answer is most likely yes. We live in a fallen world full of sin and suffering. The answer to suffering starts with prayer.

James knew that, and he ends his letter by stating the obvious. You have a Father in heaven Who loves you so much, so if you are suffering, pray often and pray hard.

Prayer isn't used as much as it can be. Often, we pray when we are in trouble. I hear all the time of people starting to pray in jail. There is nothing wrong with that as we should pray in jail, but we can also pray at all other times.

Sometimes, prayer is hard. This may be why James puts a lot of emphasis on friendship and support in his book. When you are part of a church, of a supportive community, James says to call on them and have them pray with you, support you, and help you bear your burdens. They can't help if they don't know. Prayer, and allowing others to pray with and for you is a lifeline many ignore.

You can totally trust God when He says He will respond when you call out for help. Needing help is not a sign of being a weak individual. It's just the opposite! A strong man or woman seeks help.

Daily Reflective Thoughts:

My Prayer: Lord, I need help,

Seeking help,

Day 28: Prayer of Faith

James 5:15 "And the prayer offered in faith will restore the one who is sick; and the Lord will raise him up, and if he has committed sins, they will be forgiven him."

This passage is talking about the forgiveness of sins through confession.

When you take a closer look at the passage, you see it says, "prayer offered in faith will restore the one who is sick." There are times when our sin can cause sickness. I do not believe that this passage tells us that all sickness is a result of sin, nor do I believe it is saying that all sickness can be healed. But if sin has contributed to sickness, confession and repentance is a good place to start.

Take some time to evaluate your heart, your actions, your motives. Evaluation is a great thing! Is there sin in your heart? Is there something you need to make right? Do you need to ask someone for forgiveness? Do you need to forgive someone? Is there unresolved anger you need to deal with?

Some individuals have sickness because of unconfessed sin; some may be sick because of sin and not know it. I strongly believe this is where true friendship comes into play.

Sometimes God uses others in our lives to bring these things to our attention. Take heart: Jesus has overcome sin and death, and a life committed to Him in faith is a life that overcomes!

Daily Reflective Thoughts:

My Prayer: Jesus, by faith I submit,

Committed to You,

Day 29: Confess Your Sins 1:1

James 5:16 "Therefore, confess your sins to one another, and pray for one another so that you may be healed. The effective prayer of a righteous man can accomplish much."

One Sunday, I was speaking at a small church in Northern Indiana.

The services started with a hymn, and then they asked for the public confession of sins. I was startled by the request, but the congregation was not. Over the next twenty minutes, person after person asked the congregation to pray for them as they were struggling with different sins. It was powerful.

I was reminded that day why community is so important. Many of us hide our sin; we are embarrassed and ashamed. Not at this church! They were fighting for each other, and it was refreshing.

What James is *not* saying in this verse is that the public confession of sins will forgive your sins. Only God can forgive sins (see 1 John 1:9). What he *is* saying is that together we are stronger.

We can fight better together. Together we can hold one another accountable. Together we can help each other with the struggles of sin that so easily beset us.

Another word of caution: this type of community is built over time and with much trust. Please don't walk into church next Sunday and confess all your sins in public. Build the trust first. Start small with a counselor, pastor, or friend. Then build a network of other Christians who can join you in the fight against sin.

Daily Reflective Thoughts:

My Prayer: Lord, I need help,

Trusting You,

Day 30: Pray for Each Other

James 5:16 "Therefore, confess your sins to one another, and pray for one another so that you may be healed. The effective prayer of a righteous man can accomplish much."

Pray for one another! This is not a suggestion; it's a command.

Some of the most powerful conversations I have had are with those who pray for me. I covet it. I know I need it! In community, when others know our sins and struggles, they know how to pray for us and hold us accountable.

Too often, addiction and other sins are kept private because of the associated shame and guilt. While understandable, this hiding causes far more problems and destruction in our lives and the lives of those we love.

We need open and honest communication with people of God who can intercede with and for us. Do you have a community like this? If not, it's time to get started building it. The support and connection is so important.

To those who love someone struggling with life-altering sins, and to those struggling, please don't shy away from talking about what may be seen as a tough, taboo topic. Get involved, pray, talk, intercede.

We all need this kind of community and accountability, especially when we don't know we do.

Daily Reflective Thoughts:

My Prayer: Lord, I can't do this alone,

Help me,

Closing Thoughts

Thank you for joining me on this 30-day journey through the book of James.

I know that my heart was moved as I wrote this devotional, and I hope yours has been impacted from your *30 Days in James* as well. Too often we feel like our struggles are ours alone to bear on a long, lonely journey with very little support. Take heart, my friend, that while this world may fail you, Jesus never will!

My journey in life has had some major lows and some amazing recoveries. I own my failures and sins, of which there are many, and I can only attribute my successes in life to the transformational work of Christ in my heart. I have been blessed living a life with my Savior by my side, directing my heart and steps at every turn. I want that for you! You can experience the freedom from sin, addiction, and other life-altering struggles through a relationship with Jesus Christ!

All it takes is surrender. Surrender everything - your heart and life - to Him. It's the best step you will ever take!

I would love to help you start on this journey. Please feel free to contact me through my email. Find me at BowerBrandon@gmail.com. I would love to chat about your journey and share how Christ can help set you free.

When you send an email to me, I will respond, but please be patient as it may take a little bit. But you have my promise that I will follow through as long as I have the breath to do so.

Thanks again for joining me. Be well, and I pray you will find freedom through Christ's abundant love for you!

Sincerely,
Dr. Brandon Bower

An Explanation of the Gospel

The gospel is something I was raised around. I heard it from the time I could understand and process words. My parents were faithful Christians and gave their life in service to God. The gospel, while known to me, wasn't real in my life until much later.

The author C.S. Lewis once wrote that "God whispers to us in our pleasures, speaks in our conscience, but shouts in our pains: it is His megaphone to rouse a deaf world." God used pain in my life as a megaphone pointing straight to the gospel.

I remember sitting in a police station across from my dad trying to figure out how I would talk my way out of the trouble I had just gotten myself in. Through God's gracious love for me and provision, counseling was going to be a forced part of my near future.

Dr. Allchin was the chosen counselor to meet with me. Little did I know that this older man would have such an impact on my life. It wasn't really anything that Dr. Allchin did, but who he was. As a young teen, I saw what I wanted to see... an old man who seemed rich, nice office, and a really nice car. I didn't want counseling and faked it through most of my time with Dr. Allchin. But I wanted more for my life, and this old biblical counselor had something I wanted. Stability.

So, I enrolled in counseling school. In counseling training, I met Jesus for myself. God had used the pain in my life to put me directly in the path of people who loved me, directed me, and showed me how the gospel can really change my heart.

What is the gospel? Let's start at the beginning. Mankind was created by God to be in relationship with Him. We are told in Scripture that He walked and talked with Adam and Eve and had a personal relationship with them (Genesis 3:8). Adam and Eve had it great, a relationship with the God of the universe Who loved them and met their every need.

Unfortunately, Adam and Eve wanted more. They were tempted by their hearts' desires to try and be "like God." They chose selfishly to disobey God and pursue God-like status (Genesis 3:5).

As a result of Adam and Eve's sin, relationship with God was broken; thus, all men choose to sin (Romans 3:23). Here is the good news. God wasn't satisfied with the broken relationship, so He designed a cosmic plan to save man and return humankind to a personal relationship with Him (John 3:16).

God's plan involved sending His Son to earth (1 John 4:9), Who was born human (Luke 2:7), lived a sinless perfect life (Hebrews 4), died a painful death that He didn't deserve to be a perfect substitute for us, paid for our sins completely (Hebrews 2:9), and rose from the dead conquering sin and death (1 Corinthians 15). He literally traded His righteousness for our sin.

Because of God's plan and Jesus's sacrifice on the cross, we can experience life-changing forgiveness by faith. This faith (complete trust in the Savior) is driven by love for Him and cannot be destroyed by life's troubles or trials. This life-changing faith is evidence of true salvation in your life and is the source of blessing.

There are two things you need to know: First, you need more help than you realize or can supply. Neither you, nor anyone you know, has the power to supply the help that you need.

Second, Jesus Christ is the person Who will supply that help, and if you come to Him, He will never leave you nor forsake you. There isn't much more that you need to understand than this. If you really believe these truths, your life will be transformed.

Below are some verses that will be of help for you if you want a further dive into this good news:

Romans 3:23

Romans 6:23

Romans 5:6-8

2 Corinthians 5:21

John 6:37

Romans 10:9-13

2 Corinthians 5:17

Romans 8:1

One last thought. In His great kindness and wisdom, God established a plan to help you understand and process the good news. It is through connection with others who believe this same way. We call it our church family. It is a great place to find a mentor, counselor, or just someone to help explain things to you that you may not clearly understand. I trust my friends at G3 (Gospel-Grace-Glory) to help guide you to a good church. Here is a link to good churches in your area: https://g3min.org/g3-church-network/map/

Take the step, I promise you that you won't regret it. I didn't!

Resources

Additional resources to grow your faith are listed here.

Case for a Creator – Lee Strobel
Addictions: A Banquet in the Grave – Ed Welch
Don't Waste Your Life – John Piper
Finally Free – Heath Lambert
Hell's Best Kept Secret – Ray Comfort
How People Change – Paul Tripp
Idols of the Heart – Elyse Fitzpatrick
Gospel Treason: Betraying the Gospel With Hidden Idols – Brad Bigney
Instruments in the Redeemer's Hands – Paul Tripp
MacArthur Study Bible – John MacArthur
Our Sufficiency in Christ – Dr. John MacArthur
Putting Your Past in Its Place – Stephen Viars
Slave – Dr. John MacArthur
Suffering – Paul Tripp

The Gospel of Jesus Christ – Paul Washer
The Gospel Primer – Milton Vincent
The Great Love of God – Heath Lambert
The Heart of Addiction – Mark Shaw
Trusting God – Jerry Bridges
What Do I Do Now? A Guide for Those Who Love an Addict – Dr. Brandon Bower
What Is the Gospel? – Greg Gilbert
When People Are Big and God Is Small – Edward T. Welch

About The Lighthouse

At The Lighthouse, we base our values solely on Scripture, seeking to obey and apply its teachings in everything we do.

Matthew 28:18-20 says, "Jesus came and spoke to them, saying, 'All authority has been given to Me in heaven and on earth. Go therefore and make disciples of all the nations, baptizing them in the name of the Father and of the Son and of the Holy Spirit, teaching them to observe all things that I have commanded you; and lo, I am with you always, even to the end of the age. Amen.'"

We are called by Christ to make disciples of all nations, teaching them to observe all things He has commanded. At The Lighthouse, we follow this direct command by reaching the underserved population of those who struggle with life-altering addiction and coming alongside those who love them.

It is our desire and passion to reach out to those ensnared in addiction and proclaim to them the transforming message of the gospel and the freedom that is offered in Christ. Because of our own personal life experiences, and seeing the devastating effects of addiction, we strive to minister to all within our reach through gospel-centered discipleship.

Our vision allows us to see beyond the way things are to what needs to be done to answer their cry. Though they have been ravaged by addiction, these valuable souls are ready for the gospel.

Our prayer is that you join us in furthering the gospel. If you would like to contact The Lighthouse, please visit www.lhfw.org.

Scripture Index

These Scripture verses are included

Works Cited

MacArthur, *An Introduction to James, Part 1,* Sermon given on May 11, 1986

Google definition, **Redeem**, the act of saving or being saved from sin, or evil. The action of regaining possession of something in exchange for payment or clearing a debt. To buy back, August 2023

Google definition, **Wavering**, to sway to and fro to flutter. To flicker or quiver. To shake, tremble; show doubt or indecision, August 2023

Google definition, **Double Minded**, wavering in mind; undecided. Marked by hypocrisy; insincere, August 2023

Google definition, **Confess**, admits or state that one has committed a crime or is at fault in some way. To declare, August 2023

Google definition, **Wrath**, extreme anger. Rage, fury, indignation, August 2023

Google definition, **Moral Failure**, wrong behavior; going against moral values. Sin, wrongdoing, wickedness, August 2023

Google definition, **Slander**, the action or crime of making false statements. Damaging a person's reputation with lies, August 2023

Google definition, **Guilty**, responsible for wrongdoing. A standing of guilt, July2023

Google definition, **Intercede**, to intervene on behalf of another. To pray for, July 2023

Miller, *A Praying Life* (Colorado Springs, Colorado, NavPress, 2009) Page 237

Google definition, **Prayer**, a request for help. An act of asking God, January 2023

Lewis, *Mere Christianity* (Great Brittain, Collins Clear-Type Press: London and Glasgow, 1956) Page 108

Google definition, **Humble**, a modest view of one's importance. Freedom from pride; not arrogant, June 2023

McGee, J Vernon, *James* (Glendale, California, Griffin Printing and Lithograph Co., Inc., 1983) Page 97

Lewis, *The Problem of Pain* (San Fransisco, California HarperOne 2015) Pages 57-58

Acknowledgements

To Elizabeth,
who reminds me often to "preach truth to myself."
This journey we are on has been wild and amazing.
Thanks for your support, help, and love.

Psalm 121:1-2 "I
lift up my eyes to the
mountains – where
does my help come
from?
My help comes from
the Lord, the Mak-
er of heaven and
earth."

About the Author

Brandon Bower is a passion-driven visionary with a heart to see the lost and hurting come to know healing.

Brandon Bower is the founder and director of The Lighthouse, an outreach focused on helping the hurting and broken reestablish life in the community through transitional housing for men, one-on-one mentorship, and community outreach.

Growing up in Chicago as a pastor's kid, Brandon found himself living two very different lives—one being the good pastor's kid and the other being a young, rebellious teenager running far from God. Through law-enforced counseling, God continued to work in Brandon's heart, giving him a deep passion and sensitivity toward reaching those who have and are experiencing similar difficulties.

Brandon received his Doctorate in Theology from Slidell Baptist Seminary, and his Masters in Counseling through Trinity Theological Seminary. In addition, Brandon is a Licensed Clinical Addictions Counselor and a Commissioned Addictions Biblical Counselor.

Brandon continues to share hope with individuals through one-on-one relationships, mentorship, community outreach, church teaching, group meetings, television, radio, and multiple social media platforms. Brandon served in the USA and South Africa, and has traveled abroad extensively—teaching, advising, and ministering to the hurt and broken and planting seeds of hope here and abroad.

Brandon is blessed to live this mission with his wife, Elizabeth, and their three beautiful children. They currently reside near Fort Wayne, Indiana.

Made in the USA
Las Vegas, NV
31 October 2025

33483858R00069